The **Mental** and **Physical Effects** of **Obesity**

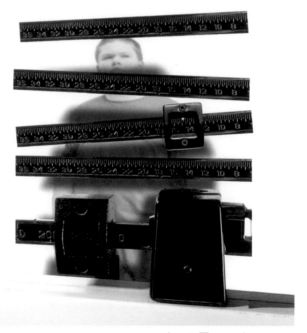

Jeri Freedman

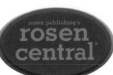

rosen publishing's
rosen central®

New York

090806

To my niece and nephew, Laura and Matthew Freedman, with love

Published in 2009 by The Rosen Publishing Group, Inc.
29 East 21st Street, New York, NY 10010
www.rosenpublishing.com

Library of Congress Cataloging-in-Publication Data

Freedman, Jeri.
Understanding obesity : the mental and physical effects of obesity / Jeri Freedman.—1st ed.
    p. cm.
Includes bibliographical references and index.
ISBN-13: 978-1-4042-1770-6 (library binding)
1. Obesity. I. Title.
RC628.F737 2009
362.196'398—dc22

2007049651

Manufactured in the United States of America

On the cover: An obese youth stands in front of a scale.

Contents

Introduction

The term "obesity" comes from the Latin *obedere*, which means "overeat" (*ob* means "over," and *edere* means "to eat"). Obesity occurs when your body stores too much fat. This leads to an unhealthy weight gain. "Unhealthy" is the key word here. Being obese is not the same as being overweight. Being overweight simply means that a person weighs more than is typical for people of the same age and height. A person may weigh significantly more than average without being obese. This is often the case with athletes, especially male athletes. When men work out, their muscles get bigger and heavier. However, the fact that they weigh more than other men of the same size does not make them unhealthy.

Standard charts defining the healthy weight for children of both genders and of different ages have been developed by the National Center for Health Statistics (NCHS). Scientifically, obesity is defined as weighing more than 30 percent over the weight defined as typical for one's age, height, and gender by standard weight tables.

A technique that is frequently used to measure obesity is the body mass index (BMI). The BMI is a mathematical formula that is used to establish what percentage of a person's weight is due to fat as opposed to lean body mass such as muscle. The NCHS developed a set of body mass index charts, which it released in 2000. The NCHS recommends that, as part of regular checkups, doctors measure a child's height, weight, and body mass index

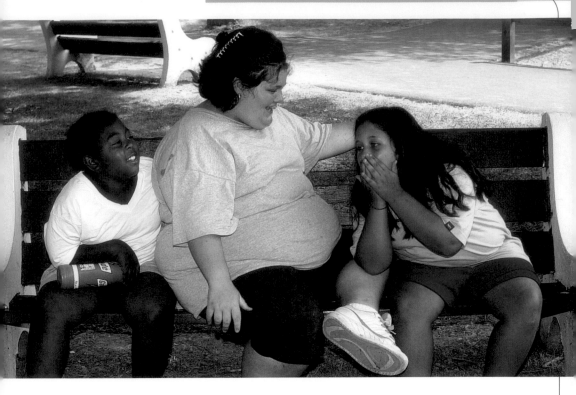

The number of obese children is increasing worldwide. The World Health Organization has declared childhood obesity to be a medical crisis.

and compare these to the charts for children of the same age, height, and gender.

In general, a BMI of 18.5 to 25 is considered healthy. A BMI of 25 to 30 indicates that a person is overweight. A BMI of 30 to 40 indicates that a person is obese, and a BMI of greater than 40 is considered morbidly, or dangerously, obese.

Being obese can lead to a variety of health problems, including heart disease, sleep problems, arthritis (inflammation of the joints), and diabetes mellitus (a condition in which the body doesn't make enough of a chemical needed to digest sugar). Experts estimate that as much as 35 percent of the population is obese today.

Obesity doesn't just affect adults. Over the past few decades, obesity has become a major health issue among children. The number of obese children has tripled in the last thirty years.

Approximately 15 percent of children are thought to be obese today. Eighty percent of obese teenagers will remain obese as adults. Obesity has led to an increase in a number of health problems in young people, including high blood pressure and diabetes, which used to be diseases that mostly affected older people. There is great concern that obesity lowers the overall life expectancy of people.

Obesity doesn't just affect the body. Obese young people are often the subjects of teasing and harassment in social situations or by other students in school. This book discusses some of the causes of obesity, its physical and mental effects, and some ways to reduce obesity and live a healthier life.

Chapter 1

What Causes Obesity?

It's common to think that people are obese because they eat too much. In truth, a number of factors play a role in obesity. Some of these factors are biological, while others are psychological (relating to the mind) or social issues. In this chapter, we'll examine some of the major factors that can lead to obesity.

WHAT HAPPENS WHEN WE EAT?

To understand why people become obese, it helps to understand how and why we store fat. You may know that the term "calorie" is linked with food. You may have heard that a cookie may have 50 calories or a can of soda may have 200 calories. But what is a calorie?

Scientifically, one calorie is the amount of energy required to raise the temperature of 1 gram of water 1 degree Celsius. Simply put, the number of calories in a food is the amount of energy the body can produce from it. The following are the daily calorie requirements for young people at different ages (the higher number is for more active people):

Age	Calories Girls	Calories Boys
9–13	1,600–2,000	1,800–2,200
14–18	2,000	2,200–2,400
19–30	2,000–2,400	2,400–3,000

When you eat, the food is broken down and carried by the bloodstream to your body's cells. In the cells are tiny organs called mitochondria. The mitochondria are like tiny furnaces. Using the oxygen you breathe, they burn the nutrients in food, and thus produce energy that the body uses to fuel its functions.

Just like an automobile, you need a certain amount of energy to keep your body going. How much energy you need depends on your level of activity. Even at rest you need some fuel to keep your basic bodily functions working. When you think, you need energy for your brain cells. When you move, you need energy for your muscle cells. As with an automobile, how much fuel you need depends on how far and how fast you're going. And that's where a problem can arise.

When you consume more calories than you need for your current activities, the excess calories are stored as fat. It is necessary to have some body fat because it insulates the body and acts as a shock absorber. However, having too much fat can

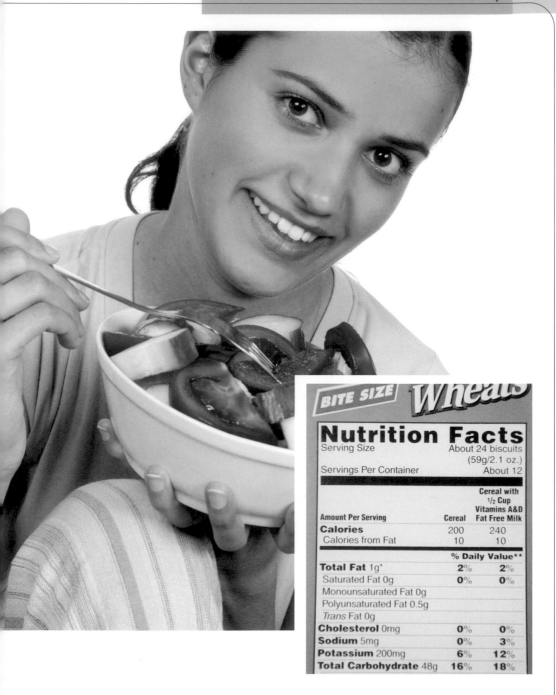

Nutrition Facts		
Serving Size		About 24 biscuits (59g/2.1 oz.)
Servings Per Container		About 12
		Cereal with ¹/₂ Cup Vitamins A&D Fat Free Milk
Amount Per Serving	Cereal	
Calories	200	240
Calories from Fat	10	10
	% Daily Value**	
Total Fat 1g*	2%	2%
Saturated Fat 0g	0%	0%
Monounsaturated Fat 0g		
Polyunsaturated Fat 0.5g		
Trans Fat 0g		
Cholesterol 0mg	0%	0%
Sodium 5mg	0%	3%
Potassium 200mg	6%	12%
Total Carbohydrate 48g	16%	18%

One way to avoid eating more calories than you need is to eat foods that are low in calories. Nutritional labeling tells you how many calories a food contains.

9

lead to health problems. In modern times, it is easy to eat many more calories than we need. The following sections explain some of the reasons why.

EVOLUTION

Human beings have been on Earth for about three million years. We have had easy access to food, through modern agriculture and modern food markets, for only a couple of hundred years. What does this mean? For most of human existence, food was scarce—often very scarce. People often faced long periods when food was hard to find.

Therefore, throughout most of human history, it was to our advantage to be able to eat as much as possible when food was available and store the excess calories for times when food was not available. Those who could store excess calories the best were often most likely to survive. Today, in our society, when a lot of food is almost always available, there are two qualities that incline us to obesity: the ability to store calories very well, and the craving for the types of foods that have the most calories and produce the most energy—fats and carbohydrates (sugars).

GENETICS

Genetic information is passed from parents to children via chromosomes. Chromosomes are threadlike elements found in the nucleus (center) of cells. Chromosomes are made of the chemical compound deoxyribonucleic acid (DNA).

Humans have twenty-three pairs of chromosomes. We get one of each pair from our mother and one from our father.

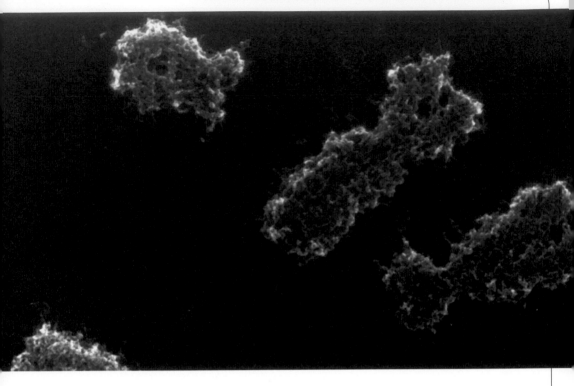

Human chromosomes, such as these seen under a microscope, carry our genetic blueprint. Our chromosomes contain thirty thousand to forty thousand genes.

Chromosomes are composed of genes. Each gene is a unique sequence of DNA. Each gene or combination of genes codes for a specific trait, such as hair color. In recent years, scientists have begun investigating a variety of ways in which genes might influence obesity. Genes involved in the following processes make it more likely that a person will become obese:

- Genes that control the sensation of hunger and satiety (the feeling of being full).
- Genes that increase or decrease the body's use of fat as fuel.

How Advertisers Lure You into Bad Choices

According to a 2004 study by the Kaiser Family Foundation, the average child sees forty thousand ads on television each year. Many of these advertise candy, soda, snack foods, and meals from fast-food restaurants. The very fact that companies spend billions of advertising dollars each year on their products shows that these companies believe their advertising influences young people's eating choices.

Several studies have shown that the amount of time children spent watching television was a good predictor of which products these children would ask their parents to buy at the grocery store. The study found that as many as three out of four products requested were those seen in television ads.

Advertising can affect children in another way. It can mislead them about the health effects of foods. In one study, 70 percent of six- to eight-year-olds believed that fast food was healthier than homemade food.

Industry publications for advertisers in the food industry have repeatedly stated that young people are a significant source of potential income because they have money to spend and they can influence their parents' choices of what to buy. Two ways that advertisers try to influence you are by connecting their product to people who seem cool, like extreme sports athletes or rock stars, and by tying in the product with characters from popular movies or TV programs. They hope that you'll eat or drink the product because it will make you feel like the person in the ad. The bottom line: Don't be manipulated by advertising.

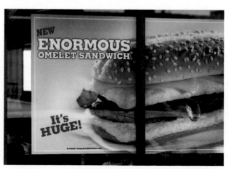

Fast-food advertising is believed to be a major contributor to obesity in America.

- Genes that increase or decrease the tendency to store body fat.
- Genes that affect the metabolism, or how much energy you need to run your body functions. How much fuel you burn in a given time to keep your body running affects how many calories you can consume before the excess is stored as fat.
- Genes that control the number of pleasure receptors in the brain. Receptors are socket-like elements to which chemicals in the body attach themselves in order to turn on or off processes in the body.

Studies have shown that identical twins tend to have similar body mass indexes, even when raised separately. Family studies have also shown that obese parents are more likely to have obese children. This is especially true of children under the age of ten. Some of this influence may be due to the environment in which they live—the behaviors of the parents may influence what a child eats. However, researchers are investigating whether factors like a preference for fatty foods and poor appetite control might be affected by genes.

A recent study by researchers at the University of Buffalo has shown that people who have fewer receptors in the brain for a chemical called dopamine, which makes us experience pleasure, eat more than people with the normal number of receptors. It appears that these people need to eat more than other people to feel satisfied.

The identification of genes that might lead to obesity is still in the early stages. Many different genes that might influence obesity are being investigated. According to the U.S. Centers for Disease

Control and Prevention, several independent studies have reported that a gene referred to as an FTO (fat mass- and obesity-associated) gene "might be responsible for up to 22 percent of all cases of common obesity in the general population." However, the exact function of the gene has not been found. Scientists are currently studying this gene to learn more.

FAST FATTY FOOD

The January 2003 issue of *Pediatrics* magazine reported a study conducted by Dr. David Ludwig, director of the Children's Hospital in Boston, Massachusetts. The study found that the amount of fast food eaten today by children ages four to nineteen is five times what it was in 1970. Since fast food is high in fats and sugar, the study suggested that it could be a factor in the increase in childhood obesity.

The study suggested that eating fast food could add as much as six pounds per year to the weight of a child. A fifteen-year study conducted by Ludwig and Mark Periera, of the University of Minnesota, examined adults ages eighteen to thirty. The results were reported in the January 2005 issue of the British medical journal the *Lancet*.

The study revealed a strong relationship between eating fast food and obesity. Eating fast food increased the likelihood of obesity, even when the researchers took into account other factors such as drinking alcohol, smoking, and level of physical activity.

In recent years, cutbacks in funding for education have forced many schools to raise money by adding vending machines that

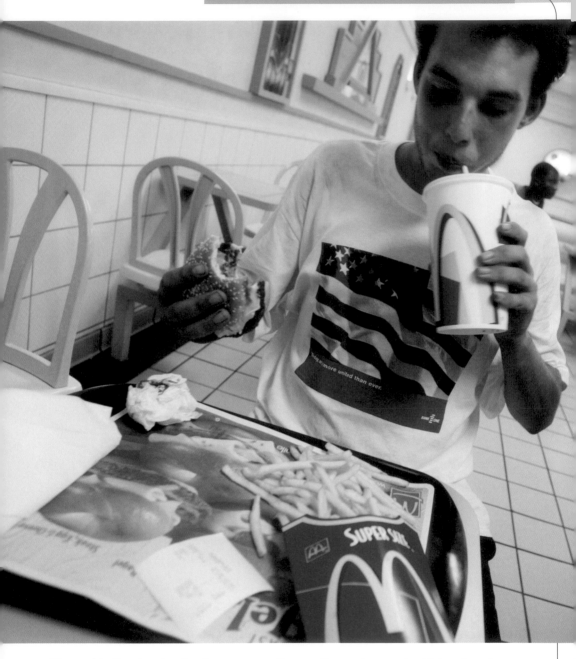

"Supersizing" makes fast food even worse for you. Researchers at the University of Wisconsin have estimated that supersizing can add as much as 73 percent more calories to a meal.

sell soda and high-sugar/high-fat snacks such as potato chips and candy. Whereas children were once limited to milk and water as beverages in school, they now can consume hundreds of calories from sugar in soda and eat unhealthy snacks at will.

LACK OF PHYSICAL ACTIVITY

The simple fact is that the more you exercise, the more energy you expend, and the more fuel you burn. Thus, getting exercise means that you will burn more of the calories you consume, and fewer will be stored as fat. It also increases the chance that you will burn stored fat. Also, exercise builds muscles, and muscles use more energy than other body tissues.

However, it is common today for many people to lead largely sedentary (inactive) lives. A 2004 study by the Kaiser Family Foundation found that children today spend on average five and a half hours per day engaged in sedentary media-based activities, including watching TV and videos, playing video games, and surfing the Internet. Studies have shown that the more time people spend watching TV, the more likely they are to be obese. This is not because TV causes obesity. Rather, people are watching TV instead of engaging in more active forms of entertainment, like playing sports or games that involve running; taking walks; riding bicycles; or other physical activities.

In addition, prior to the early twentieth century, people mainly walked to many places, including to work, to the market, and to their friends' houses. Today, we mostly rely on cars to get us from one place to another.

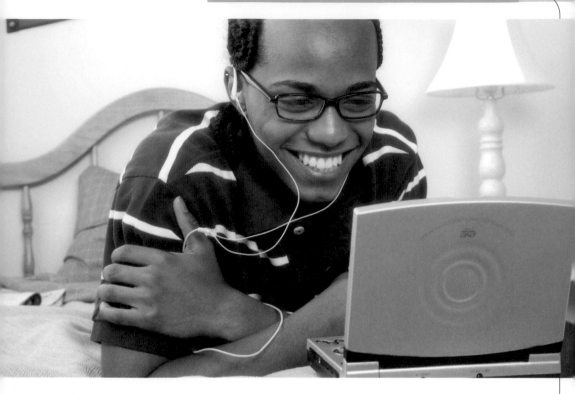

How much time do you spend playing video games, watching TV, and surfing the Internet? Spending some of that time doing physical activity instead can help control your weight.

LACK OF ROLE MODELS

Children and teenagers learn how to behave from adults. OK, you probably don't always listen to your parents. However, by and large, you develop many habits as a child by copying the things that your parents (and older siblings) do. This is true in the areas of eating and physical activity, too. The problem is that in modern society, many adults tend to set bad examples when it comes to both eating and exercise habits.

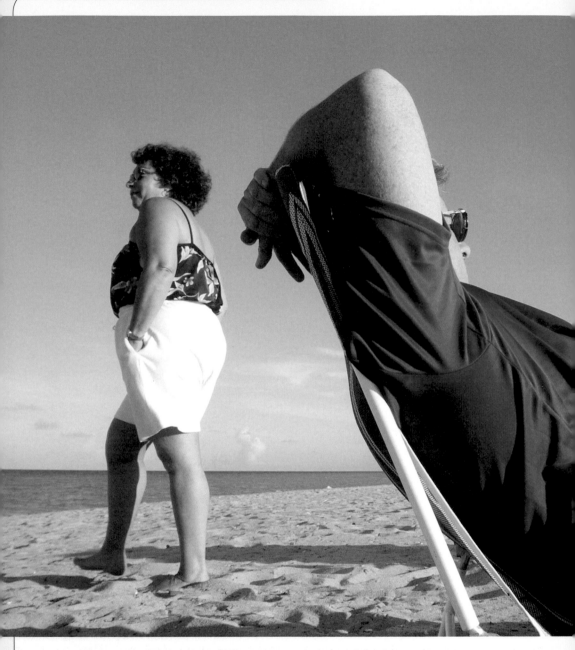

Overworked adults often engage in sedentary activities outside of work. A recent study has revealed that one in five people do work, another sedentary activity, during vacation time.

Adults in industrialized nations, including the United States and Canada, are busier than ever before, but in offices, not out in the fields doing physical labor. Two-income families have become the norm as costs have continued to rise throughout the twentieth and twenty-first centuries.

Businesses faced with the need to control costs are pressuring employees to work longer and harder. This means that more and more children have parents who are sedentary. People often arrive home from work tired, and they spend the evening watching TV or engaging in other nonphysical activities. They are forced to cram errands into weekends, and they often spend a lot of time driving from place to place to accomplish these errands. Or, they have to do work at home that they couldn't finish during the day.

For many reasons, adults often do not have the time or the energy to pursue sports or physical activities with their children. Children whose parents don't engage in physical activities are not likely to do so either. In addition, the necessity for both parents to work in order to make ends meet has had a negative impact on people's eating habits. More and more adults are bringing food home from fast-food restaurants, regular restaurants, and grocery store prepared-food departments, rather than cooking meals at home. The National Restaurant Industry Association's 2006 Restaurant Forecast estimated takeout food sales at $142.4 billion in 2006 and total restaurant food sales at $511 billion.

According to the same survey, 34 percent of the people questioned said takeout food was an essential part of their life. Prepared food is often higher in fat than food cooked at home. Children who grow up in families where adults get little exercise and rely on prepared food are likely to do the same when they grow up.

FINANCIAL PRESSURE

Although there are obese people of all income levels, a greater percentage of poor people are obese. One reason for this is that food that is high in fat and carbohydrates (sugar) tends to be inexpensive (for example, hamburgers or pasta). Food that is low in fat tends to be more expensive (such as fish, fruit, and vegetables).

Chapter 2

The Physical Effects of Obesity

Being obese puts extra strain on muscles and joints. This can lead to arthritis, which is an inflammation of the joints. People who are obese are also at greater risk for dislocating joints, especially the hips and knees. A joint is a space in which one part of the body, often a bone, is connected to another. When pressure causes a bone to move off its correct position in a joint, this is called a dislocation. Dislocation can cause a lot of pain. Carrying too much weight can also cause joints and bones to become misshapen, which can be painful and can limit one's mobility.

DIABETES

A hormone is a type of chemical produced by cells in the body that regulates a bodily process. Insulin is a hormone produced by an organ called the pancreas. Insulin

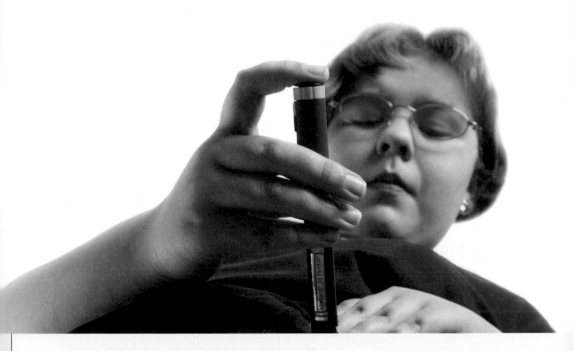

Many young people with diabetes, like this obese teenaged girl, have to give themselves injections of insulin several times a day in order to stay healthy.

is necessary to break down the sugar we eat to produce energy. Diabetes is a disease in which the body does not produce enough insulin.

There are two types of diabetes. Type 1 diabetes is an immune system disease in which the body's own immune system cells attack and destroy the insulin-producing cells in the pancreas. This type of diabetes affects only about 10 percent of the people who have diabetes.

Ninety percent of people with diabetes have type 2 diabetes. Studies have shown a close relationship between obesity and type 2 diabetes. In the past, most cases of type 2 diabetes were diagnosed in middle-aged and elderly people. However, in recent years, increasing numbers of preteens and teens have been diagnosed with type 2 diabetes.

This is bad for two reasons. First, the condition complicates the lives of young people. Diabetes must be strictly controlled with a special diet and medication, and the level of sugar in the blood must be monitored constantly. If this is not done, then crippling and other, potentially fatal, problems can occur.

Second, people with diabetes are more likely to experience problems with blood circulation, blindness, and kidney disease. As the number of young people with diabetes rises, the number of young people with these other problems will grow as well.

EFFECTS ON THE HEART AND BLOOD PRESSURE

Obesity often goes hand in hand with high cholesterol and high blood pressure. Cholesterol is a fatty substance that is used by the body to make certain hormones. It is commonly found in meat and other fats that we eat. There are two types of cholesterol: low-density lipoprotein (LDL) cholesterol and high-density lipoprotein (HDL) cholesterol.

We need some HDL cholesterol, but too much LDL cholesterol can cause health problems. LDL cholesterol sticks to the walls of blood vessels. When it builds up in blood vessels, this means that there is less space for blood to pass through, which in turn can lead to high blood pressure. Blood pressure is a measure of the force that the heart has to exert in order to move blood from the lungs, where it picks up oxygen, to the rest of the body, where the oxygen and nutrients carried by the blood are used. If blood pressure is too high, this can lead to a heart attack or stroke

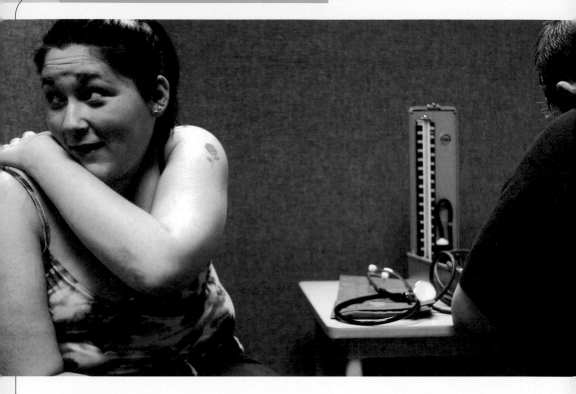

Losing weight is not easy. This young woman has entered a program that includes strict calorie control and exercise. The health benefits could add years to her life.

(the bursting of a blood vessel in the brain). Either condition can have crippling, or even fatal, effects.

GALLBLADDER PROBLEMS

The gallbladder is a small, sac-like organ located under your liver in the upper-right abdomen. It produces a liquid called bile, which helps digest fat. One of the elements that make up bile is cholesterol.

As mentioned earlier, a buildup of cholesterol is associated with obesity. When too much cholesterol builds up in the gallbladder,

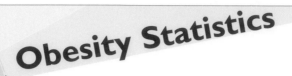

Obesity Statistics

The following are some statistics related to obesity in the United States and Canada:

- Thirty-two percent of American adults over the age of twenty are obese.
- Twenty-three percent of Canadian adults are obese.
- Seventeen percent of Americans between the ages of six and nineteen are obese.
- Eight percent of Canadians between the ages of two and seventeen are obese.
- In the past twenty years, the percentage of overweight Americans who are six to eleven years old has doubled; the percentage of overweight twelve- to nineteen-year-olds has tripled.
- In the past twenty-five years, the rate of obesity among Canadian teenagers has tripled from 3 to 9 percent.

this can lead to gallstones, which are pebble-like materials. Gallstones can block the ducts (tubes) through which the bile leaves the gallbladder. This can be very painful, and it sometimes requires surgery to fix.

OBESITY AND CANCER

A number of studies have shown a link between obesity and several major types of cancer, including cancers of the breast, colon (intestine), esophagus (the tube that runs from the throat to the stomach), kidney, and gallbladder. In 2002, forty-one thousand new cases of cancer were linked to obesity (about 3.2 percent of

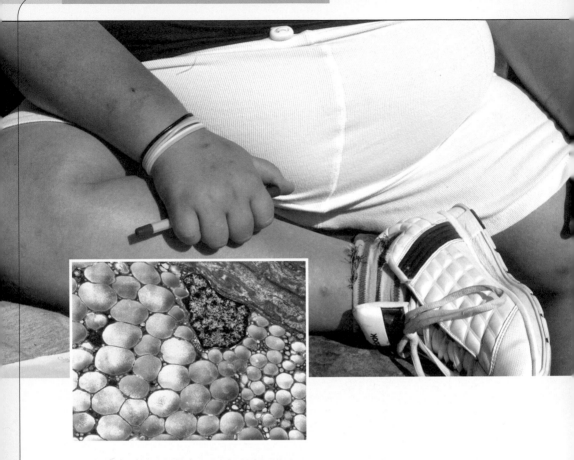

Abdominal fat is especially dangerous to one's health, since it produces hormones that affect the body. The small photo shows a human fat cell seen through a microscope.

all cases), and 14 percent of cancer-related deaths in men and 20 percent in women were linked to obesity, according to the National Cancer Institute.

In particular, after menopause (the stopping of the menstrual cycle), women who are obese are more likely to develop breast cancer. Fat tissue produces hormones. This is especially true of fat concentrated in the abdomen.

One of these hormones is the female sex hormone estrogen. After menopause, most women produce less estrogen. The fat tissue in obese women, however, continues to produce high levels of estrogen. This can lead to the development of cancer in estrogen-sensitive tissue such as the lining of the uterus and breast tissue.

Obese men are more likely than nonobese men to get colon cancer. Some studies suggest there is a link between an output of insulin and related hormones and colon cancer. Scientists do not know why obesity increases the risk of various types of cancer. However, some suspect that the increased levels of hormones put out by abdominal fat affects the tissues.

In addition to a greater likelihood of getting cancer, being obese increases the risks associated with surgery. Being obese means that a surgeon has to cut through much more tissue than would otherwise be the case. In addition, fat does not have as well developed a network of blood vessels as muscle tissue. Therefore, it is harder for the body to get an adequate amount of immune system cells to the area where the surgery has taken place, so obese people are more likely to get infections after surgery.

SLEEP DISORDERS

There is a clear link between sleep disorders and obesity. It is now known that people who are obese are more likely to have a type of sleep disorder called sleep apnea. People with this disorder periodically stop breathing during sleep. They then tend to wake up abruptly.

At one time it was thought that obesity caused sleep apnea. Now, scientists are less certain as to what is the cause and what is the effect. Studies have shown that people who don't get enough sleep are likely to eat more. Not getting enough sleep leads to a decrease in the level of a hormone called leptin that suppresses (turns off) people's appetite and speeds up their metabolism.

Lack of sleep also leads to an increase in another hormone, grehlin, which increases appetite. In addition, people with sleep apnea are more likely to be tired and, therefore, exercise less. As a result, scientists are exploring whether not getting enough sleep contributes to obesity.

OBESITY AND AGING

A large percentage of obese teenagers become obese adults. The longer you are obese and the earlier you get disorders such as diabetes or heart, lung, or joint problems, the worse their effects are likely to be as time goes on. Obesity can shorten your lifespan, so it is worthwhile to try to get your weight under control. Two studies done in 2003 found that obesity reduced the lifespan of men by five to thirteen years and the lifespan of women by seven to eight years. Be careful, though—reducing your weight too much can harm you as well. Chapter 5 provides some information on how to approach this situation in a healthy way.

Chapter 3

The Mental Effects of Obesity

O besity can have mental and emotional effects that can be just as serious as the physical health effects. The way that others see you and treat you can have short-term and long-term effects on how you see yourself and how you relate to others.

SOCIAL ISOLATION AND LONELINESS

If you are obese, you may find that you are often ignored by other kids or dismissed from their activities. You may try to put a good face on things by pretending this doesn't bother you or by clowning around. However, even people who aren't interested in the activities of popular kids find that their feelings are hurt when they are treated as though they are inferior.

Unfortunately, in our society there is a great deal of emphasis on

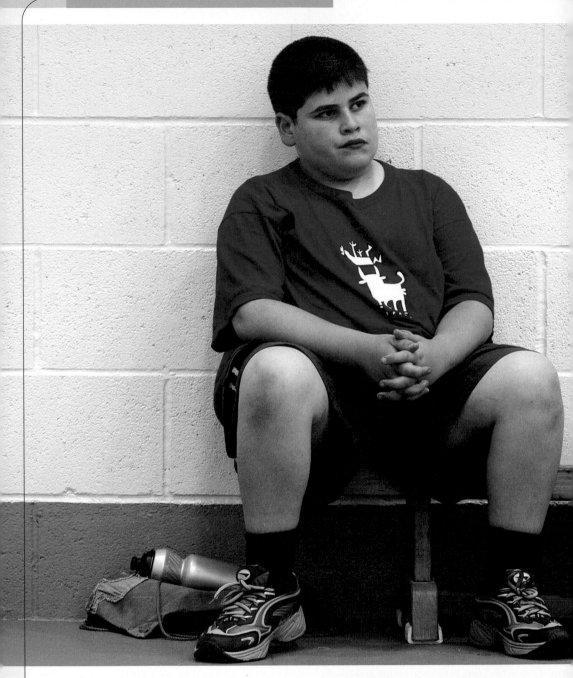

School sports are often competitive, and those who are obese are often shunned when teams are chosen, making gym a lonely and embarrassing experience.

competition. We often put too much emphasis on doing things that make us feel superior and too little emphasis on accepting people who are different. Since kids hang out in groups, not belonging to a group can make you feel isolated and lonely.

Teenagers in particular are inclined to be self-conscious and deeply concerned with what other teenagers, especially those of the opposite sex, think of them. To make matters worse, overweight teenagers are less likely to date. This is partly because they may feel self-conscious about their appearance and, therefore, shy away from people of the opposite sex out of fear of being rejected.

TEN GREAT QUESTIONS TO ASK A DOCTOR

1. Am I clinically overweight?
2. What is my ideal weight?
3. Are any of my present health problems due to my weight, and will they improve if I lose weight?
4. Where can I find a nutritionist who can help me work out a healthy diet?
5. What level of exercise would be appropriate for me?
6. Is there medication that it would be appropriate for me to take that would help me control my appetite?
7. What health problems might I develop from being overweight?
8. Is there a support group I can join to help me deal with obesity issues?
9. Are there specific types of foods that I should cut down on?
10. How much weight should I aim to lose each week?

Dealing with People Who Hassle You

Kids who are obese often find themselves being hassled by other kids. Mean kids may try to push you around physically, say things to try to embarrass you, exclude you from their group, talk about you behind your back, or post insulting comments about you in e-mails or on the Internet. Constant bullying can make you miserable.

If a bully threatens you physically, it is important to tell a responsible adult. If you don't, the bully may become increasingly violent and you could be seriously harmed. By having an adult take appropriate steps right away, you may also save other people from being harmed by that bully.

Bullies are usually insecure themselves. They cover up their insecurities by acting aggressive in front of other people. Therefore, the best way to respond when faced with a bully is to appear confident and controlled. This can often have a greater effect than getting angry, which tells the bully that he or she has succeeded in hurting you. Maintaining your self-control gives you control of the situation.

Use humor to defuse the situation. Humor often leaves an attacker unsure of how to respond. If you make the others present laugh, this puts positive attention on you and takes away attention from the bully, again transferring control of the situation to you.

After you are away from the bully, get rid of your tension by doing physical exercise or by writing about your feelings. Talking to a counselor, friend, or therapist can also help you deal with the bad feelings that a bully evokes.

People who are with a group of their friends may hassle those who are different because they think this is what their friends expect. Sometimes, talking to the person who hassles you when he or she is alone can lead to an understanding. It can be useful to talk to someone who is close to the person who is picking on you. Explain how hurtful the person's behavior is, and ask for help in getting him or her to stop the bullying. Often, a close friend will tell the person he or she is acting like a jerk.

EFFECTS ON SELF-ESTEEM

Obese young people are often subjected to nasty comments and jokes at their expense. What's worse is that they are constantly bombarded with TV shows, movies, magazines, and ads that equate being thin with being attractive and successful. Therefore, they are inclined to believe that the criticism they receive is valid and that they deserve it because they are obese. This can have a very bad effect on their self-esteem. They feel that they are both unattractive and doomed to be failures.

DEPRESSION

There is a clear link between obesity and depression. Depression is a condition of having extreme feelings of sadness and hopelessness. Studies have shown that the longer a young person is obese, the more likely he or she is to suffer from depression and other psychological conditions. A study by Jeffrey Schimmer of the University of California, San Diego, found that obese young people scored as low on tests of self-esteem as children undergoing treatment for cancer.

Feeling lonely, isolated, unattractive, and harassed can contribute to depression. However, it also appears that depression can be a cause of obesity. Depressed people often have low energy, which makes them less likely to get exercise and more likely to stay home and eat. Furthermore, depression often affects people's ability to sleep. And, as mentioned earlier, being sleep deprived often leads to more weight gain.

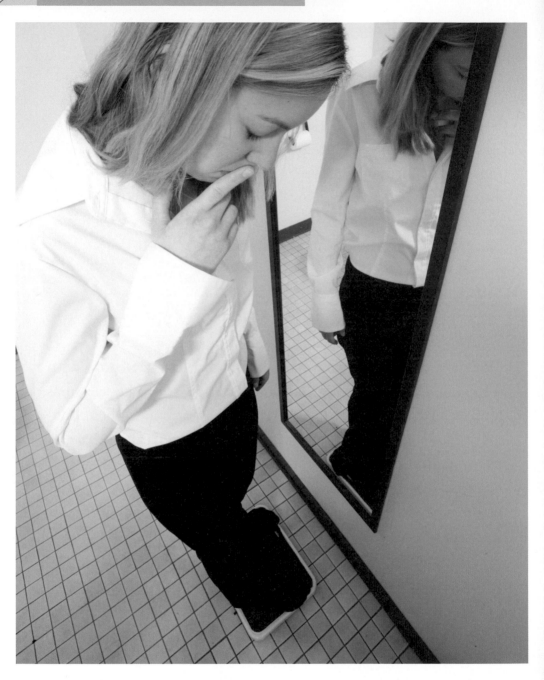

Body image is of great importance to young people. Studies have shown that girls as young as eight have learned to judge people by how they look.

EATING DISORDERS

Obesity can increase your chances of developing an eating disorder. There are physical and mental reasons for this. Being obese can lead to an obsession with weight and dieting. Too much emphasis on one's weight can lead to constant and extreme dieting that deprives the body of necessary nutrients. Too much of an obsession with dieting can lead to binge eating and bulimia. Bulimia is when a person eats large amounts of food and then makes himself or herself vomit to keep from digesting it. The stomach acid brought up in this way can damage the throat and esophagus.

An obsession with dieting can be harmful, too. Severely restricting your intake of calories can cause your body to respond in an unhealthy fashion. Often, the body becomes more efficient at drawing nutrients from food, which is in short supply. Then, if the diet is stopped, this improvement in efficiency persists, making it harder to lose weight in the future.

Another eating disorder you should be aware of is anorexia. Anorexia is a condition that causes a person to starve himself or herself. This condition can result from a combination of physical and psychological issues. Extreme dieting can lead to a loss of appetite. A person may not feel hungry, even after losing a healthy amount of weight. In addition, people who have created a mental picture of themselves as fat often keep seeing themselves that way, even after they have reached a normal weight. Anorexia can be as dangerous as obesity, sometimes more so, because if your weight gets too low, your body organs can fail and you can die.

It is important to understand that dieting by itself will not necessarily tone your body and reduce flabbiness. To have a tight

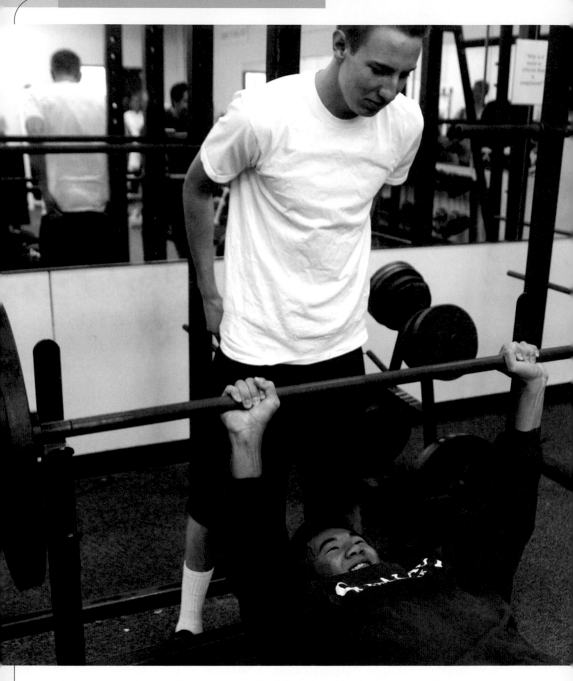

Working out is a healthy way to get in shape and lose weight. The staff at a gym can help you design a program to meet your specific goals.

and firm body, you need to exercise. You may be at your ideal weight, but when you look in the mirror, you see flesh that seems to hang loose. The way to improve the look of your body is not to diet more and hope to lose this flab. Instead, visit your local YMCA, gym, or health club and talk to a trainer on staff. That person can give you specific exercises that will build strong, tight muscles and improve the overall look and strength of your body in a healthy way.

Chapter 4

Living a Healthier Life

If you eat properly and exercise regularly, you will feel better and stay healthier longer. Remember, whatever health issues you have now will likely become greater problems as you age. Developing healthy habits now will improve your quality of life for decades to come. Even if you develop a health problem, your body will be better able to deal with the problem and its treatment if you get into the habit of maintaining a healthy lifestyle.

EXERCISE

In North America—and indeed in most of the world—many sports are seen as competitive activities. Whether it's the World Series or the World Cup, winning is what is considered more important, not having fun while doing the activity.

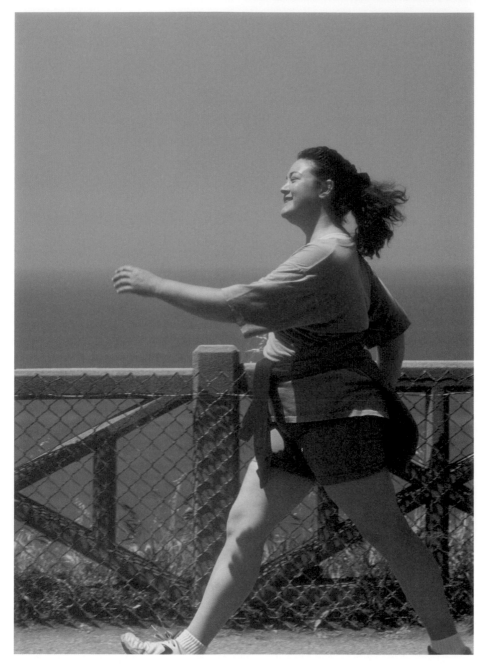

Walking is a healthy form of exercise. It can also be relaxing and improve your mental outlook if you do it in a pleasant environment.

Therefore, those who already have the fittest bodies are chosen to play again and again, while those who are overweight are discouraged from playing and are often ridiculed. This, in turn, makes overweight people hate the mere idea of participating in sports, so they are less likely to engage in physical activity.

It's important to know that there are many physical activities that (1) can be fun when played in a noncompetitive way, and (2) can be done alone or with one or two friends. Physical activity causes you to breathe in more oxygen. It can make you feel more energetic. Exercise also causes the body to release chemicals called endorphins, which make you feel good.

If you don't feel like participating in a group sport, you can take up a solitary activity such as swimming or biking. Go for thirty-minute walks. Walking for thirty minutes several times a week will improve your health without requiring you to engage in strenuous activity. You could also try a martial art such as judo, karate, or tai chi.

CHANGE YOUR RELATIONSHIP WITH FOOD

We don't just eat to survive. If we did, no one would be obese. The fact is that we use food to satisfy a variety of needs. In many cases, our relationship to food is not ideal. We eat for many reasons, to fill needs that would be more healthily addressed in other ways. Here are some of the ways we use food:

- **As a reward:** When we do well, we often reward ourselves with a treat such as candy, ice cream, or cake. One approach to healthy eating is to use nonfood

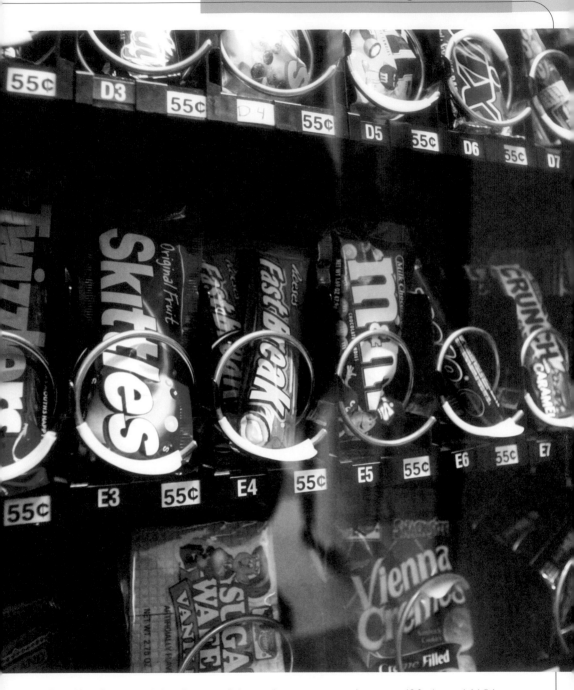

Reaching for a candy bar is one of the easiest ways to make yourself feel good. With a little thought, though, you can think of other ways to reward yourself.

rewards instead. Treat yourself to a movie or concert, a new book or CD, a trip to the mall, or something else nonedible instead.

- **To make you feel better:** When we are sad or lonely, we often turn to food to make us feel better. Research has shown that chocolate and carbohydrates contain chemicals that naturally make us feel better. Healthier approaches to feeling better include (1) talking to someone about your feelings, (2) using nonedible ways of cheering yourself up, like watching a funny movie, and (3) volunteering if you are feeling lonely. When you help out at a charity, you will meet people who are less likely to be judgmental. The others involved will value you for what you're doing, which is good for your self-esteem. In addition, you'll feel good because you're helping other people.

- **As a social activity:** We often use food as a reason to get together with our friends—going out for ice cream, burgers and fries, pizza, and the like. Socializing is important, but you can try to pick places that provide healthy offerings, or you can choose non-food-related destinations.

- **To get rid of boredom:** Often, we eat when we are bored. The body craves stimulation, and food provides it. Try to find an alternative to eating instead.

In short, eat only when you are hungry. Starving yourself is as bad as overeating, but if you find yourself eating when you are not really hungry, think about why you are eating and see if you can think of a healthier way to satisfy your need.

Studies by various researchers, including groups at the University of Toronto and Cornell University in New York, have revealed that how much we eat has very little to do with how hungry we are. They found that most overeating occurs when we do feel hungry but do not feel full either. Often it occurs when we are focused on other things, such as talking to friends or watching TV. We are not paying attention to how our body feels, and so we keep eating even though we are not actually hungry.

Myths and Facts

Myth: It's OK to eat all you want of a food if it's marked "low fat."
Fact: Many foods that are labeled "low fat" are actually very high in sugar. Excess sugar is converted into fat in the body. It's healthier to eat foods that are low in fat and sugar.

Myth: If it's served in my school, it must be healthy.
Fact: Many schools sell foods that are high in fat and sugar, like soft drinks and candy. In addition, many school cafeterias offer foods that are high in fat, such as french fries, because they think these will appeal to young people.

Myth: The best way to lose weight is not to eat.
Fact: Skipping meals or fasting is likely to make your body use calories more efficiently, thereby making it harder to lose weight over time. You will also be deprived of the nutrients you need to stay healthy.

Chapter 5

Losing Weight

According to the National Cancer Institute, if you are obese, losing even 5 to 10 percent of your weight can make you healthier. However, the goal is to achieve the right weight and do it in a healthy fashion. The previous chapter provided some tips on healthy exercise. This chapter provides some tips on eating right. It also provides some information on treatments for serious cases of obesity.

ARE YOU REALLY OBESE?

Before you decide that you need to lose weight, you should establish whether you are actually obese. The incorrect way to judge if you are obese is to look in the mirror and decide you're not pleased with your appearance or to ask your friends if they think you look fat. Consult with a professional such as your

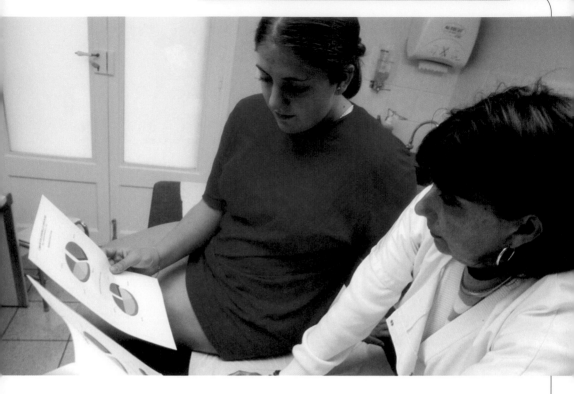

A teenager consults with a nutritionist at a center that helps obese teens. Professionals such as this can help you design a healthy plan to reach your ideal weight.

family doctor. This professional can use objective measures to see how your present weight compares with the normal weight for people of your height, gender, and age.

Your primary care physician can evaluate your weight or can refer you to a professional who can do so. If you do need to lose weight, your doctor can also refer you to a nutritionist, who can help you work out a proper healthy diet. Also, your doctor can make sure that your obesity is not the result of a medical problem.

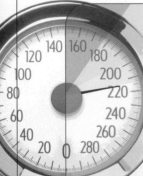

What the Labels Really Say

Here's what the terms found on the nutritional labels of processed foods can really tell you.

- **Carbohydrate:** A compound in food composed mostly of sugar.
- **Fiber:** An indigestible structural component of food that aids digestion. It is desirable to eat a moderate amount of fiber from sources such as vegetables and whole grains.
- **Hydrogenated vegetable oil:** A form of vegetable oil that has been processed to give it a long shelf life; it is difficult for the body to break down and is high in trans fat. It can clog your arteries, leading to high blood pressure.
- **Protein:** The component in food that contains the basic building blocks necessary to build body tissues. Food high in protein and fiber and low in fat and carbohydrates is generally good for you.
- **Saturated fat:** A form of fat that raises low-density lipoprotein (LDL), or bad, cholesterol.
- **Servings:** The first thing you should do is check the serving size. Is it a realistic serving? If you are going to eat half a bag of chips or a whole can of soup, multiply the components on the label by the number of servings you're actually going to eat.
- **Sodium, or salt:** Too much salt in your diet may lead you to retain water, which your body needs to dilute to a safe level. This may increase your blood pressure.
- **Trans fat:** A type of dietary fat that can increase bad cholesterol and reduce good cholesterol without providing any nutritional benefit.
- **Unsaturated or polyunsaturated fat:** A type of fat found in healthy vegetable oils such as olive and canola oil, and in fish. It is recommended that you eat 25 grams per day of this type of fat in order to supply your body with the dietary fat it needs.

GOOD AND BAD DIETS

Don't diet—eat right. The fact is, if you are overweight but you eat the right foods in the right amounts (in addition to exercising), you will most likely lose weight. The key to a healthy diet is to feel full while eating things that are high in nutritional value and low in fat and sugar. Here a few more points to keep in mind about dieting:

1. Become familiar with the food pyramid recommended by nutritionists at the U.S. Department of Agriculture (USDA). According to the food pyramid, you should get the majority of your calories from vegetables, milk, whole grains, and fruit, with smaller amounts from meat and healthy oils, like olive oil, which supply a little bit of fat.

2. Set a realistic goal and time frame for your weight loss. Your goal should be to get down to a medically healthy weight, and you should plan to lose weight slowly—for instance, a pound or two per week. Trying to lose large amounts of weight quickly by indulging in fasting or "quick fix" diets is not only unhealthy, but it is also unsuccessful in most cases.

3. Try to avoid eating foods full of "empty calories"—foods such as candy and cake that have a lot of sugar and fat but few nutrients. Foods that have empty calories can add weight, but they provide little nutritional benefit.

4. Don't go to dietary extremes. Diets that tell you to eat no carbohydrates or all protein, or encourage you to

follow any other bizarre formula for losing weight, are likely to deprive you of necessary nutrients. Besides, they will be impossible for you to maintain over the long run. The fact is, you need a little of most elements in food, even fat and carbohydrates. Just don't eat too much of them!

5. Practice portion control. Eat a little of a variety of foods. Then stop and see if you feel full. If you do feel full, stop eating. You need a well-balanced diet to be healthy, but many people eat two or more times the amount of food necessary at mealtime. That extra food becomes stored fat.

6. Work with a friend or a group. As with many things, it's harder to reach a goal by yourself without the support of others. If you have a friend or friends who want to lose weight, or if you know a teacher or counselor who would be willing to sponsor an after-school weight-loss support group, work together.

Losing weight in a healthy manner can improve your self-esteem as well as your physical health because it demonstrates that you can take control of your life. And that builds confidence for dealing with other issues you will encounter in life.

MEDICAL SOLUTIONS TO OBESITY

Medical approaches to treating obesity are most commonly used in very severe cases of obesity. In those cases, a person is so obese that his or her health is at risk; therefore, significant weight loss is required. Medical approaches to treating obesity

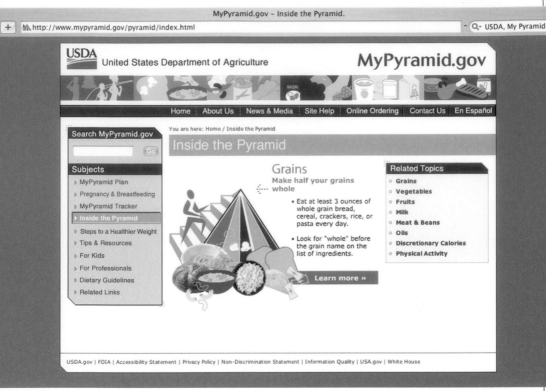

The MyPyramid Web page on the USDA Web site (www.MyPyramid.gov) can help you create a personalized plan for healthy eating based on the food pyramid.

fall into two categories: medication and surgery. The medications most often used are aimed at either controlling the appetite or reducing intestinal fat. An example of a medication that suppresses the appetite is Meridia. It is recommended for people who are more than 30 pounds (13.6 kilograms) overweight. An example of a medication that works by reducing the intake of food is Xenical. It keeps the digestive system from digesting about 30 percent of the dietary fat eaten. It is recommended for people who are more than 30 pounds (13.6 kilograms) overweight or whose body mass index (BMI) is more than 30.

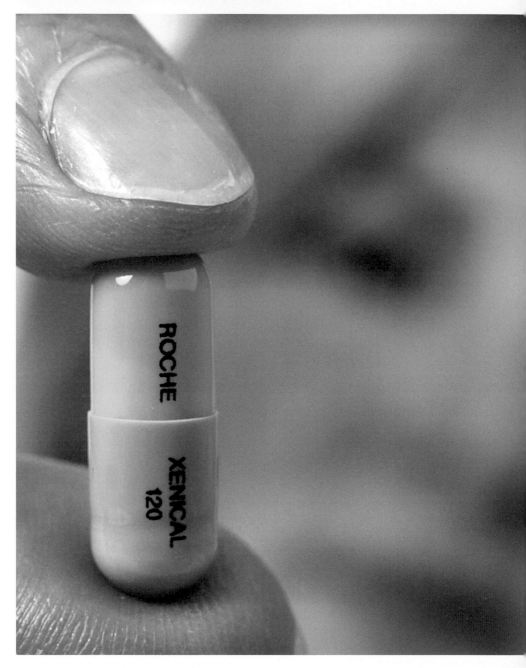

Xenical is an antiobesity drug that keeps the body from absorbing some of the fat that is eaten. It also helps reduce the amount of LDL cholesterol in the blood.

Surgery for weight loss should be used only as a last resort because of all the possible complications. The most common form of weight-loss surgery is aimed at reducing the size of the stomach. The idea is that if the stomach is smaller, a person will feel full sooner and will, therefore, eat less. In a common form of this surgery, a band is placed around part of the stomach in order to reduce its size. The advantage of this type of surgery is that it is reversible.

Another surgical approach to treating obesity is the gastric bypass operation. In this case, the length of the intestine is reduced so that food will spend less time in the stomach and less of it will be absorbed into the body. Stomach surgery still requires the patient to control how much food he or she eats because it is possible to stretch the stomach. However, it makes it more likely that the person will feel full with less food, thereby making it easier for him or her to control food intake.

RESEARCH INTO OBESITY

Recently, scientists have been researching the genetic basis of obesity and the possible ways to control it. Much research in this area has been done with mice. Recently, scientists at Johns Hopkins University in Baltimore, Maryland, found that eliminating a gene for a compound called myostatin from mice produced leaner, healthier mice. Myostatin limits muscle growth, keeping the mice from developing excessively large muscles. The mice without the gene grew more muscle and less fat.

It is not practical to remove a gene from people, and the side effects of doing so are unknown. However, this research opens up the possibility of developing medications that could be used

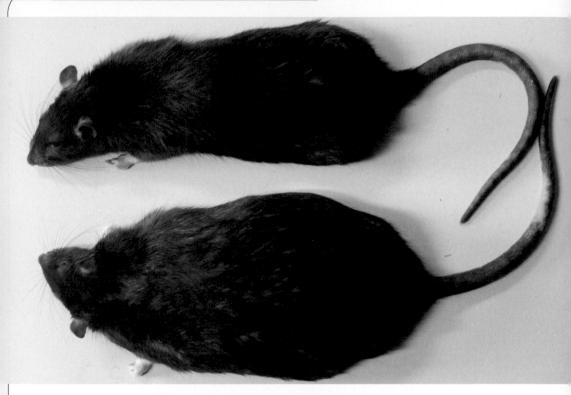

Shown here are a mouse of normal weight *(top)* and an obese mouse *(bottom)*. Studying such differences in animals provides scientists with valuable clues as to the nature of obesity in people.

to block the activity of myostatin on an as-needed basis to encourage more lean muscle growth and less fat storage.

Recently, researchers found a link between certain types of obesity and bacteria that live in the digestive system. Bacteria that live in the digestive system help us break down food, allowing us to use the nutrients it contains. In studying obese and skinny mice, researchers found that the thin mice had a greater amount of a kind of bacteria called *Bacteroidetes*. The researchers then examined a group of overweight people and found that they, like the obese mice, had less of this kind of bacteria. They instructed these people to go on a diet. As they became thinner over the next year, the proportion of *Bacteroidetes* in their digestive systems increased. However, researchers still have to determine the significance of their findings. Do the bacteria influence weight gain, or does weight gain change the population of bacteria?

Another approach is aimed at eliminating the negative health effects from obesity. Scientists recently established that feeding obese mice an extract made from red wine reduced the bad health effects of obesity. Obese mice that were fed the extract, along with a high-calorie diet, had less heart disease and diabetes and 30 percent fewer obesity-related deaths than the mice that were not fed the extract. However, there is still much to be discovered through research, and there is little doubt that we will continue to learn more about the causes of obesity and how to control its effects in the years to come.

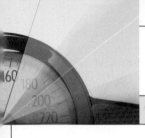

Glossary

anorexia An eating disorder in which a person seriously restricts his or her intake of food.

arthritis Inflammation of the joints.

body mass index (BMI) A scientific formula used to calculate how much fat a person carries.

calorie The amount of energy required to raise 1 gram of water 1 degree in temperature.

carbohydrate A compound found in food that consists mostly of sugar, which the body burns for energy.

cholesterol A fatty substance produced in the body or consumed in food; it can clog the arteries if too much of it is present.

chromosome A threadlike structure found in the center of cells; it contains genetic information.

depression Extreme feelings of sadness and hopelessness.

dislocate To move a bone out of its proper position in a joint.

esophagus The tube that runs from the throat to the stomach.

evolution The series of changes that take place in an animal or environment over time.

gene A segment of a chromosome that contains the code for one trait.

genetics The study of inherited characteristics and the material that transmits them.

hormone A chemical in the body that regulates a specific body function.

lipoprotein *Lipo* means "fat," and "protein" refers to a basic compound that makes up body tissues; a lipoprotein is a combination of these two elements.

menopause When a woman stops getting her period.

metabolism The physical processes that take place in the body.

mitochondria The tiny organs in cells that burn nutrients to create energy.

satiety A feeling of satisfaction or fullness.

sedentary Inactive; sitting a lot and getting little exercise.

shelf life How long food will last before spoiling.

sleep apnea A sleep disorder in which a person periodically stops breathing.

stroke The bursting of a blood vessel in the brain.

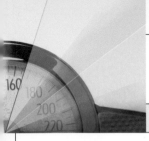

American Council for Fitness and Nutrition
P.O. Box 33396
Washington, DC 20033-3396
(800) 953-1700
Web site: http://www.acfn.org
The American Council for Fitness and Nutrition provides the
latest information on research into fitness and nutrition to
help people lead healthier lives.

Canadian Obesity Network
Royal Alexandra Hospital
Room 102, Materials Management Centre
10240 Kingsway Avenue
Edmonton, AB T5H 3V9
Canada
(289) 238-9148
Web site: http://www.obesitynetwork.ca
The Canadian Obesity Network is a source of news related to
obesity in Canada.

The Obesity Society
8630 Fenton Street, Suite 918
Silver Spring, MD 20910
(301) 563-6526

Web site: http://www.naaso.org

The Obesity Society provides information, including a variety of fact sheets, on the health effects of obesity.

Rudd Center for Food Policy and Obesity

309 Edwards Street

Yale University

New Haven, CT 06520-8369

(203) 432-6700

Web site: http://www.yaleruddcenter.org

The Rudd Center for Food Policy and Obesity is an organization that offers data on obesity, the latest news related to obesity, and school surveys.

Shaping America's Youth

Academic Network, LLC

120 NW 9th Avenue, Suite 216

Portland, OR 97209-3326

(800) 729-9221

Web site: http://www.shapingamericasyouth.org

Shaping America's Youth is an organization devoted to providing information on programs around the country that help young people increase their levels of physical activity and improve their nutrition.

Weight Watchers

11 Madison Avenue

New York, NY 10010

(212) 589-2700

Web site: http://www.weightwatchers.com
Weight Watchers is a valuable source of support and information
on how to lose weight the right way.

Web Sites

Due to the changing nature of Internet links, Rosen Publishing
has developed an online list of Web sites related to the subject of
this book. This site is updated regularly. Please use this link to
access the list:

http://www.rosenlinks.com/uno/mpeo

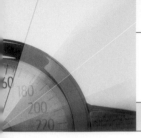

For Further Reading

Esherick, Joan. *Clothing, Cosmetic, and Self-Esteem Tips: Making the Most of the Body You Have*. Broomall, PA: Mason Crest, 2005.

Gay, Kathlyn. *Am I Fat? The Obesity Issue for Teens*. Berkeley Heights, NJ: Enslow Publishers, Inc., 2006.

Hunter, William. *Genetics: How Genetics and Environment Shape Us: The Destined Body*. Broomall, PA: Mason Crest, 2005.

Hunter, William. *Medications and Surgery for Weight Loss: When Dieting Isn't Enough*. Broomall, PA: Mason Crest, 2005.

Ingram, Scott. *Want Fries with That? Obesity and the Supersizing of America*. Danbury, CT: Franklin Watts, 2005.

Jukes, Mavis, and Lilian Wai-Lin Cheung. *Be Healthy! It's a Girl Thing: Food, Fitness, and Feeling Great*. New York, NY: Crown Books for Young Readers, 2003.

Libal, Autumn. *Fats, Sugars, and Empty Calories: The Fast Food Habit*. Broomall, PA: Mason Crest, 2004.

Owens, Peter. *Teens: Health and Obesity*. Broomall, PA: Mason Crest, 2005.

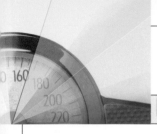

Bibliography

Ashworth, Carolyn. *Defeating the Child Obesity Epidemic.* Dallas, TX: P.S.G. Books, 2005.

Associated Press. "Study: Red Wine Extract Makes Fat Mice Healthy Again." FoxNews.com. Retrieved October 5, 2007 (http://www.foxnews.com/story/0,2933,226821,00.html).

CBS News. "Fast Food Linked to Child Obesity." Retrieved October 5, 2007 (http://www.cbsnews.com/stories/2004/01/05/health/main591325.shtml).

Centers for Disease Control and Prevention. "About BMI for Children and Teenagers." Retrieved October 5, 2007 (http://www.cdc.gov/nccdphp/dnpa/bmi/childrens_BMI/about_childrens_BMI.htm).

Centers for Disease Control and Prevention. "Obesity and Genetics: A Health Perspective." Retrieved October 5, 2007 (http://www.cdc.gov/genomics/training/perspectives/files/obesedit.htm).

Endocrine Society. *The Endocrine Society Weighs In: A Handbook on Obesity in America.* Retrieved October 5, 2007 (http://www.obesityinamerica.org/links/HandbookonObesityinAmerica.pdf).

Food Processing magazine. "Restaurant Industry Sales Expected to Reach $511 Billion in 2006." Retrieved October 5, 2007 (http://www.foodprocessing.com/industrynews/2005/584.html).

Greenfieldboyce, Nell. "Fat Bacteria in Human Guts Tied to Obesity." NPR. Retrieved October 5, 2007 (http://www.npr.org/teplates/story/story.php?storyId=6654607).

Johns Hopkins University. "Muscle Gene Influences Fat Storage in Mice; May Be Target to Prevent or Treat Obesity and Diabetes." Retrieved October 5, 2007 (http://www.hopkinsmedicine.org/press/2002/FEBRUARY/020227.htm).

Kaiser Family Foundation. "The Role of Media in Childhood Obesity." February 2004. Retrieved October 5, 2007 (http://www.kff.org/entmedia/upload/The-Role-Of-Media-in-Childhood-Obesity.pdf).

McDowell, Natasha. "Obesity's Effect on Lifespan Calculated." *New Scientist*. Retrieved October 5, 2007 (http://www.newscientist.com/article/dn3246.html).

Rim, Sylvia. *Rescuing the Emotional Lives of Overweight Children*. Kutztown, PA: Rodale, 2005.

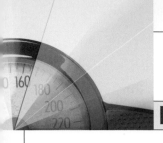

Index

About the Author

Jeri Freedman has a B.A. degree from Harvard University. For fifteen years, she has worked for companies in the medical field. Freedman is the author of more than twenty young-adult nonfiction books, many of them published by Rosen Publishing. Among her previous titles are *The Human Population and the Nitrogen Cycle*, *Hemophilia*, *Lymphoma: Current and Emerging Trends in Detection and Treatment*, *How Do We Know About Genetics and Heredity*, *Everything You Need to Know About Genetically Modified Foods*, *Autism*, and *Applications and Limitations of Taxonomy in Classification of Organisms: An Anthology of Current Thought*.

Photo Credits

Editor: Nicholas Croce

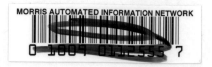